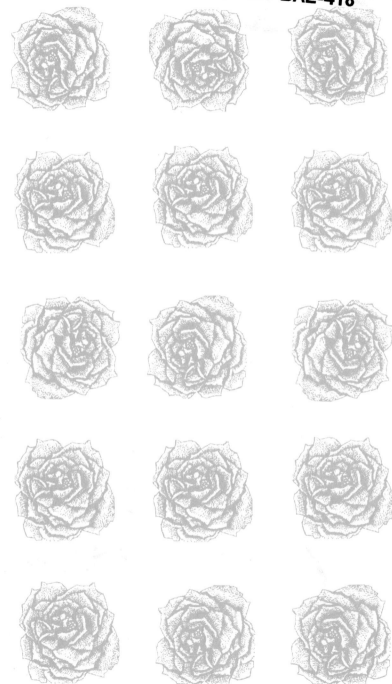

# The Life Within

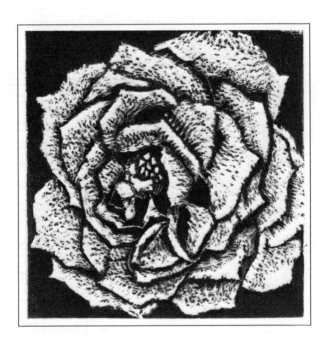

# The Life Within

## Celebration of a Pregnancy

by

# Jean Hegland

Illustrations by

### Gayle Hegland

Humana Press • Clifton, New Jersey

Excerpts of earlier versions of several chapters of this book have appeared in
*Spiritual Mothering* (The Fourth Month), *The Doula* (The Second Month), and
*A Writer's Reader* (The Fourth Month).

Library of Congress Cataloging-in-Publication Data:

Hegland, Jean.
       The life within : celebration of a pregnancy / by Jean Hegland.
            p.    cm.
       ISBN 0-89603-196-9
       1. Pregnancy.    I. Title.
       RG525.H415   1991
       612.6'3—dc20                                    90-46690
                                                       CIP

For my mother,

**Virginia Hegland,**
*née Thompson,*

*and for my daughters*
**Hannah Virginia Fisher**
**and Tessa Alma Fisher,**
*each née a Riddle*

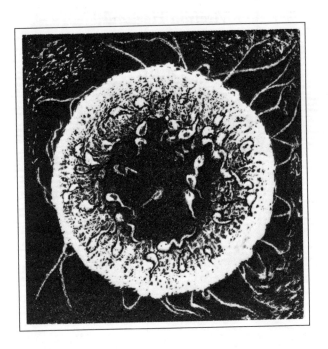

# The First Month

*The one unifying, incontrovertible experience shared by all women and men is that months-long period we spent unfolding inside a woman's body.*

**—Adrienne Rich**

I do not know when the child I am carrying was conceived. There was nothing to mark that moment, nothing to distinguish it from any of the other moments that I have lived. It was a time like any time, ordinary or special for its own reasons, lost, as soon as it passed, in the jumble of memory, remarkable only in retrospect, for in that instant, a baby was begun.

Those who study such things know that human conception occurs when a microscopic sperm travels through the cavernous reaches of the vagina, past the narrow cervix and empty uterus, and up into the convoluted tunnel of a fallopian tube, there to be absorbed at last by an ovum ninety thousand times its weight—and smaller than a speck of dust. That happens as long as two days after the coupling that set the sperm in motion, and when it does, it happens imperceptibly. There is no twinge, no omen, no shift in the world to announce its event.

This month-old embryo was conceived without my knowledge, despite my efforts to avoid it. My only consent was that of my femaleness, my fleshiness, those ancient instincts that urged me to mate, and the compliance of my own body, the ready ovum, the waiting uterus, the wash of hormones, and the rich blood willing to sustain this little mite. By the time my urine revealed its presence to me, this creature had been growing for three weeks. Hundreds of times heavier than when it began, its body was already the size of a typewritten comma, and a primitive heart was sputtering in its chest.

I think it is always rare that we are able to witness the events that change our lives. The phone call in the night, the tidal wave, the telegram, all announce things that began as we were lifting a fork to our mouths, sweeping a floor, setting a bowl of apples on the table. Even the sun's light is old by the time it reaches us. Still, I mull back over the days when this conception must have occurred, sifting through the details that compose my life, trying to reconstruct, to remember what I never knew, hoping to discover among my doings that moment of beginning. In that lost second something happened that seems more momentous than even my own breath and blood and digestion, and I long to know exactly when that instant was.

The ancient Egyptians believed that the circumstances surrounding a woman's conception could influence the nature of the person who resulted, and fifteenth century Europeans were warned that at the hour of conception a woman should not look upon monstrous things, for fear that what she saw would shape her child. It does seem as though that instant could affect the future, and I find myself hoping this conception was a tiny moment of epiphany, a second when I fit well inside my skin.

Perhaps I was dreaming when those two cells mated, curled skin to warm skin against this new creature's father, our own vigorous instincts sated as we nuzzled each other in our sleep. Or maybe this little wad of life began as I was waking, stretching beneath the flesh-hot sheets in the first gray light. Maybe I was laughing when it happened, dancing naked in the kitchen while the morning coffee brewed. Or maybe I was dressed and driving to town, following my own musings as my car droned on down the barren freeway. But perhaps if I were only folding the laundry, or signing the mortgage check, or asking Douglas to pass the salt, that moment was auspicious enough for this beginning, for it is such moments that are the substance of a life.

In a way I am glad this happened without my knowledge, just as I am glad that my bone marrow produces blood, and my gut absorbs food, and my lungs strip oxygen from the air I breathe without my conscious effort. It is a relief that biology can take care of itself, that there are parts of my life beyond my ken or control.

And yet even if the way I lived that instant cannot affect the life that—with luck—will come of it, still it seems that such a moment deserves ceremony, celebration, or maybe simply the awe that observation brings, as when we catch sight of the first green shoots huddled beneath the old snow's crust, and the dailiness of our lives halts for a moment in veneration.

And now I find myself longing to remember what we have all forgotten, what the journey begun in that instant is like. I wish that I could migrate back through the red hum of my own mother's womb, could return to the mystery from which I started. Like a film run in reverse, so that the lily is sucked back into its bud, and the ocean reclaims its waves, I would like to follow myself to my beginning.

But even that would not be far enough, for then I would like to go beyond myself, to pass through my inception, to be spit out unconceived on some other side, and still to keep on traveling, back through my simian past, back to the first reptile who thrust a shelless gob of breathing flesh from her startled womb, and then beyond that unhatched birthling until I reach at last the form-less, gathering gases of the stars.

When I look to myth to learn about begin-nings, I read again the stories of those who lived closer to our origins than we do. According to the

Navajo, it was a giant named First Woman who created humankind. Long ago, when the world was young, she spread two blankets of mist upon the ground, and on each blanket she laid many things—white shells for bones, abalone shells for toes and fingernails, darkness for hair, sky waters for tears, lightning for tongues. Then, with the help of the winds and the Sun, she gave form and motion to those assembled bits of the world, and men and women arose from the mists.

The Chinese said that the Goddess Nu Kua fashioned humankind from a lump of yellow clay because she thought that the earth, that pleasure garden the God P'an Ku had created out of his own body, seemed lonely. And the Flat-head Indians said that the first people, who were crafted of mud, were made because Old Coyote was lonely, because he wept, and had no one to talk to. I like those stories, like to think we were formed from the earth itself, formed to relieve loneliness, and I wonder whether the first living microbe that science says we came from didn't appear in the primal ocean because the water wept, and longed for company.

But in both myth and in the stories that science tells, there is always something that precedes the beginning. There is always Chaos, or Love, always a primordial atom, a protogalactic cloud, an ocean or a god alone in the lostness of unordered time, always a witness to that moment when the atom bursts, or the cloud collapses, the waters part, or the song is heard, and the world begins. So it seems that beginnings have always eluded us, receding just as we try to grasp them, leading us past the conception of a child, the origin of a species, past the creation of an earth, a galaxy, out beyond the inception of the universe itself, to where the atmosphere is too thin, the distances too vast for our tiny, human minds.

Still, it is not easy to abandon this search for beginnings, not easy to live with the thought of the past expanding behind me to infinity, and so I would like to give this child an arbitrary start. Let me say this baby was really conceived thirty-five hundred million years ago, when, adrift in an empty sea, the first molecule managed to reproduce itself. Let me say that in that second all the conceptions of this world took place, unobserved, unremembered, but celebrated as long as life continues on this planet.

Perhaps conception and birth are important to us not so much because of our excitement about beginnings, but because of our satisfaction with continuings. The Yoruba of Guinea said that each baby is the reappearance of one of its forefathers, who has come back to dwell once more among the living, and in eastern Siberia, Koryak parents used to announce a baby's birth by proclaiming, "A relative has arrived," for they believed that each person comes into existence when the Supreme Being sends an ancestor's soul to inhabit yet another body.

So it might be that parents and children are related many times, connected not only in this life, but by a web of lives gone by. I like the notion that we are not only our children's parents, but also their progeny, and I find myself wondering which, of my own dead, might be refleshing itself inside me.

Surely this pregnancy connects me with my past; even the replications of DNA are a sort of reincarnation, and my ancestors will live on in the chromosomes of this child's cells, and perhaps in its gift for music, or its taste for pickles, or the corn-flower blue of its eyes.

Once, in the bottom of a cluttered drawer I found a roll of film so old I could not remember when I had exposed it. I had it developed and when I saw the image those forgotten negatives contained, I borrowed a friend's darkroom, and in that humid, chemical blackness, I fumbled through water temperatures, exposure times, test strips, slid a blank sheet of paper into the eye-stinging developer, and gasped as my dead father's face rose from that slosh like a smiling ghost. Perhaps this pregnancy is like that, so that even now, on an empty surface in a dark room, a familiar image is ascending once more to life.

Once upon a time, there was a woman who wanted a child more than anything else in the world. And so, after much sorrow and yearning, she pricked her finger—or consulted a crone—or planted a flower, and her heart's desire was granted. That's how the stories begin. But when I first realized I might be pregnant, I reacted not with the joy I had always expected I would feel, but with denial, resentment.

9

I waited for my period to begin, certain that I had miscounted the days, certain that it was simply late. I didn't quit drinking wine or taking aspirin for three days after I finally admitted to myself that I might have conceived. The first day I still couldn't imagine that it might really be true, and the second day, along with my disbelief, there came a kind of rebellion. I felt trapped, tricked into something I had not yet chosen. By that evening I had decided to quit drinking alcohol until my period started—after all, I did want to be pregnant sometime soon; not drinking wine would be good practice for when I was. But when I woke the next morning with a brutal headache and an eight o'clock class to teach, I took two aspirin, reasoning that aspirin couldn't possibly hurt an embryo that didn't exist. Besides, I hadn't asked for this child; if it insisted on coming now, it would have to face the consequences.

That night as we lay together in bed, I told Douglas that my period was a week late, and watched his delight numbly, knowing how happy I should be to be pregnant by such a man. But I felt miserable, bullied, crowded, not by a baby, but by biology itself, by some sort of inhuman principle, some force that had suddenly, absolutely changed my life in a way I had not yet chosen.

The next day Douglas brought home a drug-store pregnancy test, and I tried to feel excitement as we studied the tubes of clear liquid, the plastic vials, and the little purple tablets like the ones I remember using to color Easter eggs when I was a child. That night I dreamed I was happy about being pregnant, and the next morning as I peed into the kit's plastic cup, I wasn't sure what I hoped the test would show.

Together Douglas and I added three drops of yellow urine to the lavender fluid we had mixed, and then we watched as it faded to palest gray. "If the liquid changes color," read the instructions, "you can assume you are pregnant."

Then together we left the house to walk by the river in the bright morning sun, stumbling, giggling, assuming I was pregnant, our arms around each other as we tried to readjust our plans for the coming summer, for work, for Christmas, tried to imagine ourselves as parents, and yet were still unable to grasp what that gray liquid meant, were still unable to do more than shiver and grin.

This was not the first time or place in which a woman has examined her urine to divine her fate. Thirty-three hundred years ago, the Egyptians wrote that if a woman's urine was cloudy, it meant that she was pregnant. Hippocrates said that the urine of a gestating woman was different from other urine, and well into the eighteenth century, European women would water certain seeds—lentil, wheat, or barley—with their urine, and then watch to see whether the hormones of pregnancy would germinate the grain.

I was not thinking of those other women as I watched my urine reveal what I could not yet know about myself, but later, after our walk, I realized I felt more connection with them than with the crumb in my womb. I thought of those hundreds of generations of women, each bent over her bowl of urine, her pot of seeds, each desperate or simply curious as she searched for the signs of her fertility, seeing the future fork abruptly out in front of her— one way if yes, another if no—hoping, perhaps, that the power of her desire could cause the seeds to germinate or halt their growth. And then I thought of all the women who, like me, had raised their heads from their search, and pressed their hands blindly to their flat bellies, wondering what it was that they contained.

But it is only for me, and not those women who have already borne their mysteries, that I haunt libraries and bookstores, and fill our house with medical texts, books of folklore, embryology, anthropology, mythology. It is only for me, and perhaps for the creature inside me, that I begin to study what people have believed, feared, hoped, or learned about human gestation, this ordinary miracle, this simple marvel, this first fact of life.

Embryologists say the odds were against this little berry from the beginning—from before the beginning—just as the odds were against its father and me, against its grandparents, and their parents, and on and on back in a widening net of chance. At the moment each of us was conceived, any one of hundreds of millions of other people might have been started instead. And if our parents had been tired that night, or too eager for each other to wait until evening, someone else would have been the result, and we, who are so solidly alive, would never have been imagined.

It is a grand mixture of precision and fluke, an intricate series of chances that mark our beginnings. Three hundred and sixty million sperm are released at once. At the rate of three inches an hour, they swarm through the vagina, struggle through the cervix to the uterus, and wander up the two fallopian tubes, only one of which might contain a ripe ovum. Of the hundreds of millions that begin the trek, only a few thousand will ever reach the ovum—if there is one—and of those final thousand, only one will ever blunder against it, and then, with the help of the ovum itself, will bore its head inside, and mate its twenty-three chromosomes with the twenty-three the ovum happens to contain. When those forty-six chromosomes finally align, a creature the world has never known is suddenly described in the infinite, eloquent, and exact language of DNA. In that moment, chance gives way to the inevitability of genetics, for there then exists a single cell poised to grow precisely in accordance with its genes.

That first cell is called a zygote, and that is how we each began—the twinkle in our parents' eyes might have produced anybody. But once luck yields to that particular coupling of chromosomes, the shape of our fingernails, the scent of our sweat, and the time at which our hair will begin to gray are determined. The characteristics that depict us are set in motion.

All this takes place in a landscape as weird as anything Dali or Dr. Seuss might imagine. Medical photographs show that our internal selves are not the solid or shadowy places we sometimes think them to be, but instead are fantastic gardens of lush texture, and startling color. Beneath the wrinkled elephant skin of a testicle, the tubules that produce sperm cluster like rosy sea anemones. And deep in their secret darkness, fallopian tubes as lavish as O'Keeffe flowers stand ready to suck newly released ova past their feathery white petals and down their crimson throats.

An ovum itself looks like a solitary planet, aloof and glowing as a moon, around whose vast and pitted surface sperm butt and thrash like tiny, animated pins. And the zygote that results from the coupling of moon and pin is glossed with the fragile sheen of mother-of-pearl and shaped like a fried egg. It is an entity as improbable as all that comes of it.

After the zygote rests for a day and a half, it begins to cleave. Cleave means both 'to divide' and 'to adhere to', and that paradox is an apt description for the cohesion of multiplying cells. The zygote doubles its chromosomes and then splits in half, giving rise to two identical cells that cling together, and, half a day later, themselves divide, each giving rise to two more cells, until in a few days, a tiny ball like a cluster of pomegranate seeds has formed, and the zygote has become a morula.

Like the snowball that begins the avalanche, the morula tumbles back down the fallopian tube and into the uterus, all the while dividing, changing, growing larger and more diverse, until a day later it has been transformed to the hollow ball biologists call a blastocyst. The blastocyst implants itself in the rich soil of the womb with a violence that belies its tiny size. It roots into the compliant uterine flesh like a foxtail seed, gorging as it goes on the blood it spills. Once buried, it flattens, grows a fluid-filled membrane to surround itself, and then lengthens, folds, its edges fusing to become a chubby tube, an embryo.

Then comes heart, and spinal cord, and gut, all primitive, all bulging and shifting like a rose opening in a time-lapsed film, all arising out of that speck of protein that was two cells, that became one, that doubled and divided, transforming from one thing to another as wildly and exactly as objects in a magician's show, where rabbits become scarves that become tulips and then coins, in a perfect, dizzying succession of change. And so these organs, these basic bits of human being appear like rabbits out of nowhere—out of the intention of the universe—and a new creature takes shape.

Zygote to morula to blastocyst to embryo— such unfamiliar, inhuman names for our beginnings. But that is what we are risen from, more truly than mud or monkeys or Adam's rib. Still, it all seems magical, impossible, or possible only as myth is possible, as metaphor to describe a mystery that will always remain intact. I might as well have been fertilized as the goddess Hera was, by the wind. I might as well have become pregnant by eating the flesh of a golden-scaled fish, or by drinking water into which a star had fallen. I can as easily believe that I am pregnant on moonbeams.

The seventeenth-century naturalists and lensmakers who first examined the world with their newly made microscopes studied semen and found that it contained minute whip-tailed creatures, all wriggling with life. When they sketched what it was they thought they were seeing, they drew a miniature person huddled in the head of every sperm.

It is no wonder those early embryologists looked through their crude and miraculous microscopes and drew what they did. Imagine looking at the fluid that caused babies through a tool meant to expose the secrets of the universe, and seeing nothing human, so that the microscope did not bring the world closer to human comprehension, but sent it reeling beyond our grasp. If there was nothing human about sperm, where did humanity come from? What was it that filled a woman's belly? How did a father beget his children?

The word 'conception' can mean the formation of either a zygote or a thought, and an old meaning of 'embryo' is that which is still idea. For me, this baby is still only the idea of a child. It is an interesting theory, a pretty fancy, but certainly not a fact. This pregnancy is still as remote as the stars, still as hard to believe in as the mites that I am told spend their microscopic lives in the jungle of my eyelashes or the cavernous reaches beneath my toenails.

In Siam it was thought that before she conceived, a woman first dreamed of her child-to-be, and in Australia, the Aborigines said that every child starts its life in its father's dreams. It makes sense to me that we begin as dream, and only later are our dream-selves cloaked in flesh.

It is a dream, a grand act of imagination on the part of the cosmos that the thing accreting in my womb could ever be a human being. After thirty days of growing, this speck of tissue is now three thousand times heavier than it was when it began, and still it is less than a quarter of an inch long, a frail, transparent blob, with a spine curved like a prawn's and a bulky head bent over its newly beating heart. Featureless, limbless, it looks like a miniature monster from some terrible late night movie. It has gill slits on either side of its eyeless head, a yolk sac that trails from its middle like a collapsed parachute, and a stubby tail that curves towards its bulbous, gaping face.

Little minnow, little sparrow, little mouse, it is a creature not yet human, which can become nothing else.

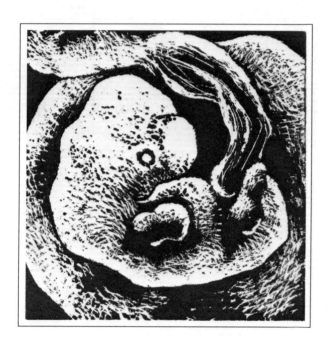

# The Second Month

*In the course of responding to influences the embryo
itself is changed so that it responds slightly differently
to the next stimulus. In this respect, embryonic
growth is similar to other creative processes.*

**Harold D. Swanson**

Human Reproduction, Biology and Social Change

In the beginning was the Word...and the
Word was God, says the Gospel of St. John, and
when that God spoke, his words incarnated a world.
According to the Nez Perce, before people arrived
upon the earth, animals enjoyed the power of
speech, but once human beings came, the animals
all fell silent. Our language is still one of the gifts
that separates us from the rest of the creatures on
this teeming planet. Other animals—dolphins,
whales, chimpanzees, bees—use patterns of sound
to communicate, but their languages lack the rich
variety, the delicate subtlety, of human speech. We

23

alone of all creatures are talkers, and of all the worlds on this earth, ours is the only one whose parts are named, as if, for us, the words themselves had made the world real.

This little blister will be born into a world of names, a world shaped by speech. Even in the womb, it is immersed in language, for as soon as it can hear, it will listen to all my talk, and by the time that it is born, it will be able to recognize the cadences and rhythms of its native tongue. Even now, when it is still no larger than a pea, it is preparing for its worded world. Its tongue, jaw, and palate have begun to form; its brain, which is now almost as large as the rest of its body, is growing more complex, so that someday it, too, can think in symbols, learn names, use language.

In some cultures this guppy would not be named until it could laugh up into its father's face, or until it could speak for itself. Here, we will name it as soon as it is born, but already its father and I have given it a name for the next eight months, a womb name. I think that we have named it to make it real to us. That which has made its presence known only by changing the color in a test tube of urine now has a name, and so it seems more tangible, closer to us than it did before.

We've taken to calling it Riddle. In ages past, a riddle solved could save a life, win a kingdom, or conjure a god. These days riddles are thought of as little more than nursery rhymes, but even so, the answer to a riddle can still startle us into seeing the world afresh, suggesting the essential mystery, the marvelous strangeness of an object as familiar as a candle flame or a cloud, an event as ordinary as the coming of a child.

A riddle is a pastime, a trick, a quest. It is the dark saying of a prophet, the deadly question that only a hero can answer. "Say what I mean, say who I am," demanded the haunting riddle-songs of the medieval Anglo-Saxons, and they told of creatures who wept as they consumed their mothers, or who were pregnant without conceiving.

If we are ever to know its answer, each riddle requires that we suspend our usual ways of thinking, that we approach it with all the imagination, intuition, and wit that we possess, and then that we tinker, play, and dream, allowing solutions to suggest themselves out of that clutter of clue and hint.

So, too, we must attempt to decipher this Riddle with our whole selves open, receptive to all that we can learn about what it means and who it is.

But there are also riddles that have no answers. They are the riddles that neither science nor philosophy can ever solve, the unfathomable enigmas of how and why, the riddles that will endure no matter how precisely we learn to crack the code of DNA, or to describe the stuff that holds the universe together, no matter how close we come to the divine. Einstein wrote about the "great, eternal riddle" of this world, and I think it is that riddle we have named our Riddle after. I think we've chosen to call this creature Riddle in order to remind ourselves of the limits of solutions, of the holiness that resides in mystery. I think we've called it Riddle to remind ourselves that even after it is born and we know its sex and the color of its eyes and hair, even after we know its name, we will never be able to say all that this Riddle means and is.

Riddle, now that you have a name, I find myself addressing you as though you could already understand my words, as though you, who reside in my womb and share the products of my blood, could also live in my mind and share my thoughts. I find myself thinking of you, who are privy to my life in a way that no one has ever been, as I used to think of God when I was a child, as an unseen, constant presence in my life, who was with me when I went to the bathroom, who knew my thoughts as I thought them, but more than that, who understood the bad and delighted in the good. Little Riddle, I think of you as being as wise as God used to be, and still, I know I am only talking to myself when I use your name; you are no more aware of me than a narcissus bulb is aware of the thawing soil it sends its roots into.

Even so, I want to know you. I feel the gardener's urge to brush back the earth and inspect her crop. I try to imagine you, Riddle, floating within me, weightless, implacable, silently growing toes, making a liver for yourself, sprouting wisps of ribs to curve over the darkness of your embryonic gut, changing shape like a tadpole, a caterpillar, a cloud, unfolding like a Chinese paper pellet that blossoms into a flower when it is placed in a bowl of water.

One of the riddles a teacher of Zen might ask his students in order to help them understand

27

the riddle that we live is, "What was your original face before you were born?" I ask that question now, not of myself, but of the Riddle growing inside me, as I study a photograph from an anatomy text captioned, "Human fetus at 40 days."

Like the sight of my own blood, it fascinates and disturbs me, that anonymous fetus, that luminous ghost, that waxy Kewpie doll, with its thick white trunk, its tiny, trailing legs, and its hands budding fingers like the fingers on a baseball mitt. The front of its head is horrible in its blandness. Noseless, chinless, with a lipless mouth and lidless eyes, it is a face as expressionless as a fish's face, sightless, selfless. I feel faint at the thought of such a thing inside me.

I try to imagine that monstrous face, those fixed eyes gazing blindly into the darkness I contain, that gaping hole which may someday become a mouth washed in the fluid it is creating around itself, and I shudder, and none of this seems real, seems possible. Human beings cannot begin like this. That series of bulges cannot be the original face of a creature who can pose itself such a question. My imagination recedes, folds back on itself, squirms away from the conundrum, while deep inside me, the face I cannot imagine is acquiring a new shape.

Sometime during this month, this bit of a child, this baby grown to the size of a peanut, will begin to move, to flail its stubby hands and stretch its delicate legs. I know those first, tentative stirrings are simply reflex actions, performed without effort or sensation, but still, I wonder what it must be like to bend a brand new elbow, to wiggle freshly made toes, and I find myself remembering that first morning each spring when my mother finally let me go barefoot, how the flesh of my soles contracted in green joy against the chilly grass.

And then there are the thousands of things that could go wrong, that may have already gone wrong, so that even after all these months of gestating, the life within me will never gain human shape, and I will give birth to something sad or frightening, or someone who cannot partake of living as easily as I do.

Last summer I found a fledgling swallow sitting so motionlessly in the grass beneath the oak tree that only its black bead of an eye convinced me it was living. It watched my approach with the dispassionate patience of the helpless, suffered me to scoop it into my cupped palm like a drink of water. It was so slight, that as I held it, my hand felt buoyed by its tiny weight, and I was suddenly aware of the crude loudness of the quiet afternoon, of my own blustering monstrosity.

That swallow must have flown once—or tried to. It must have taken to the air along with its nestmates, but while they toddled into flight, it had plunged to the ground beneath its nest, there to await starvation or a passing cat, for although one of its wings was fine and strong, the other was only a stub from which curled a few useless wisps of feather.

It was a cruel biological joke—a one-winged swallow—an unlucky roll of the chromosomes, perhaps, or perhaps the result of human beings' passion for toxins. But whatever the reason, the reason didn't matter. That bird was doomed before its hatching to a single tumbling fall. Never would it play, as I have seen other swallows play, a game of breezy catch with a straw of wheat. Never would it dart and swoop for insects in the golden air of a summer's evening.

I am haunted by that swallow these days, and by all the other deformities I have seen, heard of, all that I can imagine. I remember again and again a basement room in the small-town nursing home where I went looking for work as a teenager. It was a room filled, that spring morning, with a leafy light that flickered from the window well as if filtered through clear, deep water. Against the walls of that green-lit room were three huge cribs, and in each crib was a human woman, her face empty, her arms and legs contracted against her body, so that she lay curled into herself like a giant fetus, silently enduring the whole unalleviated weight of her life.

In her crib, each woman was as anonymous as an egg, and yet as I left that still, green room, I knew that each one of them must have had a name, that her features must have resembled someone's, that she must have broken someone's heart when she grew and grew and did not change.

I remember those women often. And I am haunted by other things. I think of monsters, of the half-human things that fill our nightmares, the children born too twisted or incomplete to survive, the blobs of distorted and misbegotten flesh in the clinical photographs of the books I read, or the pitiful things in the tabloid headlines, those thrilling horrors that remind us how fragile we are, how lucky we have been to escape such darkness.

I think of the living children that make me look away to keep from staring as I pass them on the street, the child whose limbs didn't grow, or whose spine failed to close, the baby with the huge head. I think of blindness, of deafness, of idiocy, and of the more subtle mistakes, of the child who can't learn, the baby who can't metabolize its food, the one who can't feel pain—and I panic. There is so much that can go wrong.

Each dividing cell, each growing organ must follow the four-million-year-old plan exactly—for the first time. There are no second chances. There is no going back, no catching up, no fixing mistakes. If the bones in this creature's hands haven't lengthened by now, it will never be able to grasp; if the chambers of its heart haven't formed, it will never be able to sustain its own life. Ordained in the moment of conception, reenacted in each splitting cell, this child-to-be fleshes itself out, growing inexorably towards what it will become, without my knowledge, beyond my control.

And yet both science and folklore say that the womb is not as private a place as it would seem, that one moment of inattention or ill-luck can distort a lifetime. The Malaysians thought that if a pregnant woman shot an animal in the eye, her child would be born blind. In Nigeria it was believed that if she caught sight of a monkey, her baby would be born more ape than human. American colonists said that a woman was risking the shape of her unborn if she sat with the dead, or was frightened by a snake, a wolf, a wildcat. In renaissance France it was believed that what a woman thought or how she sat could cause her to give birth to a monster.

The list goes on, a multicultural catalog of the ways a woman's experiences and actions, desires and fears can shape the flesh and spirit of her unborn: if she looks at the moon, her child will be a lunatic; if she craves strawberries, her baby will be born with the mark of her craving etched upon its skin; if she curses, her baby will be a freak; if she trips on a grave, her child will be clubfooted; if she is scared by a cripple, her infant will be crippled; if she is startled by a hare, it will have a cleft palate.

We have been told to avoid eclipses and madmen, spicy foods and wild animals, sex, heat, and too much sleep. We have been told that an imperfect child revealed our sins, our hungers, our angers, or infidelities, or that such a child was given us as an omen, a fairy's prank, the Devil's curse, a lesson from God.

More recently we have been warned about Thalidomide, radiation, rubella. We have been told about nutrition and exercise, and what the Chinese knew a thousand years ago, that the child of a tranquil mother is calmer, brighter, and weighs more at birth. And so I drink milk for the sake of this creature's bones, eat protein for its mushrooming brain. I avoid alcohol, aspirin, and stress, and yet those all seem like paltry measures, too mild to ensure the shape and senses of a child.

The folklore of pregnancy seems more real to me, with its placid explanations for what went wrong, and its elaborate rituals for avoiding trouble. I would perform sacraments and fairy tale trials to assure that this Riddle will be born quick and strong and human-shaped. I would spin straw from gold, would travel to the earth's end to steal an apple from the tree of life, if only I could win the promise of a perfect child. Still, I know I must content myself with simpler measures, and with those that have no certainty—with exercise, wholesome food, and hope.

Child, I think you are complicit in all this, too. The Aboriginal Australians believed that each mother is chosen by her unborn baby. In Nigeria it was thought that before birth all people select their own destinies. And now embryologists have discovered that it is the fetus itself that stimulates and directs at least some of the processes of its growth. In another week or so, you will move your brand new tongue out of the way so that your palate can fuse above it. Already you have turned the flesh along the embryonic tube of yourself into a nervous system; those nerves have caused your limbs to move, and those first movements have set your muscles growing. A few months from now, those same nerves will kindle your dreams, and those dreams will incite the neurons of your brain, until you have wired yourself with the ten trillion connections of action and understanding.

I like to think that you are now in the process of creating yourself, you, who demanded squatter's rights to my womb, who dug yourself into my living flesh, and there began to construct your own. In the midst of my life you are making yours, and I wish you the joy and courage of all creators as they shape their intentions and their terrors and their dreams.

But don't think that once you have built lungs that can bear the harsh weight of the air, and hands that can grasp, and a gut that can turn seeds, leaves, and flesh to flesh, bone, and power, that you are done with your work. You will never be done with the process of creating yourself, and if you ever think that you are, you will be betraying that tiny, blind larva you once were.

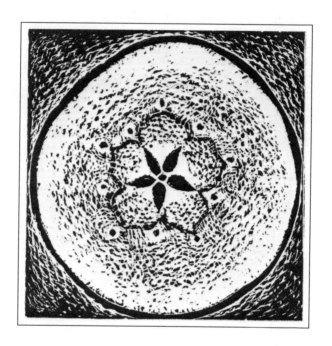

# The Third Month

*The Almighty shall bless thee with the blessings
of heaven above, with the blessings of the deep
that lieth beneath, with the blessings
of the breasts and of the womb.*

**Genesis 49: 25**

By now Riddle has grown to the size of my thumb. No longer a grotesque embryo, it is a creature with a human face and body—a fetus. The photographs show that it is a lovely, frail elf of a child, smooth and precious as a netsuke carving, glowing like ivory, like polished alabaster, with a skin so transparent its newly-formed organs darken it like shadows, and a face as sweet as a Buddha's or a Madonna's.

Those photographs remind me of the photographs I have seen of the earth itself, in which our sapphire of a planet floats serenely against the black backdrop of the universe. A three-month's fetus in the globe of its amniotic sac seems a similar jewel adrift in a similar darkness, a heavenly body at home in the infinite.

In their story of creation, the Cupeno Indians said it was Coyote who came into the world first, issuing forth from a sack suspended in the void. When Riddle arrives, it too will emerge from a sack, the rosily transparent membrane of its amniotic sac. In an earlier time, if an infant were born with a shred of that membrane still clinging to its head, it was considered a charmed child, for it was thought that such a caul could endow its owner with prescience or eloquence, or serve as a love charm, or save a drowning man at sea.

Now this creature swims in a sea of its own making. Like life itself, which both science and myth claim began in the deeps of the ocean's womb, water is this Riddle's primal element. Far from the weathers and blows of its mother's world, it cavorts in the warm comfort of amniotic fluid, and its fresh-made muscles grow strong in buoyant weightlessness. It breathes, drinks, and pees into that ocean, and so accustomed is it to the saline stuff that although a newborn will choke reflexively on fresh water or milk, it will inhale salt water like air.

40

But even after this fish has been landed, it will still be a watery being, still awash in the fluids that flow constantly through its cells, still drawn to the roar and slosh of the seas. Water is so fundamental to our earthly lives that, across time and around the world, it has played a role in the ceremonies we've used to commemorate a baby's birth. From the natives of North America to the peasants of rural Japan, from the ancient Druids and Norsemen to contemporary Christians and Hindus, we humans have used water to name and bless and welcome those who have left their amniotic oceans to join us on this sea-blue planet.

In his mother's body a man knows the universe, in birth he forgets it, says the Jewish proverb, and it does seem as though this one were in touch with a knowledge the rest of us have lost. In the photographs a twelve-week-old fetus looks as though it were contemplating its place in the cosmos or pondering its own creation as it drifts into being. Placid, remote, it seems so complete and self-contained that I am always surprised to remember that this philosopher is a freeloader, dependent entirely upon what it can mooch from my blood.

For inside its amniotic sac, its umbilical cord connects our Riddle to its placenta like an astronaut to his spacecraft or a deep sea diver to her boat. A placenta is a weird, dense pudding of an organ, just thicker than a beefsteak and roughly round as a dinner plate. On one side, the pale cable of umbilical cord rises from it like a tree trunk from a rooty tangle of blood vessels, and on the underside, those veins have thinned to tiny capillaries that entwine with the capillaries in the wall of my uterus. There, this fetus and I communicate in a language that precedes desire, the language of diffusion, so that its needs are met, molecule by molecule, before it knows them. There, its blood rushes constantly to meet mine, to strip it of its lode of oxygen and nutrients, and give me in exchange carbon dioxide, uric acid, wastes.

A fetus's placenta is its first stomach, its first lung. Of all other organs, only a brain requires as much raw energy for its tasks. A placenta is a philosopher's stone, performing the alchemy that transmutes blood to food, and I wonder whether it might not be the legendary Tree of Life itself, for from that rooted bough we all have flowered.

Born of the same cell that gave rise to it, Riddle's placenta is its genetic twin, its only companion in its first home. The Semites said a placenta was sister to the baby it had nourished, and rural Malaysians thought that if a baby smiled for no reason, it was because it was playing with its older brother, the ancient, invisible spirit that inhabited its placenta.

Of the hundreds of cultures in this world that anthropologists have been able to study, ours is one of only a handful in which placentas are disposed of as if they were trash. In Nigeria a baby's placenta will be planted fondly beneath a banana stem, and the resulting tree named for the child whose afterbirth nourished them both. A Yoruban infant's placenta is buried beside its father's house so that it will always yearn towards home, and in Okinawa it is said that a newborn will be happy if it laughs as its placenta is being dug into the earth. This child's placenta will be discarded without observance soon after it is born, and yet we should remember that odd sponge fondly, for there Riddle and I came as close to mingling as two corporeal creatures ever can.

We should remember, too, the thread by which it now clings to life. After it is born, and the cut stump of its umbilical cord sloughs off, this baby will be scarred forever with the pretty pucker of its navel, a remembrance of the communion it once took from my blood. There are cultures in which, when the dried stem of an infant's cord sloughs off, it is the signal for a feast, and there are other cultures in which the stump itself is saved as a memento or a medicine or a charm.

Here, we will consider that wizened scrap neither relic nor magic, nor will any ceremony accompany its cutting. The Mbuti pygmies say only one of its father's arrow blades can sever an infant from its placenta, and the Siriono of Bolivia believe that the father himself should cut his newborn's umbilical cord, so that if he is away when his baby is born, its cord must remain intact until he returns. But here we will clamp and cut our Riddle's cord almost as soon as it chokes air, for once that twist of flesh has ceased to pulse, we think it is as useless as an appendix, or an empty cupboard, or a disconnected phone. For us, cutting its cord will be not a ritual, but a chore, a task as simple as cleaning a hen or mending a shirt, though it seems the heart must surely cry out 'bless this cleaving' to the casual hand that holds the scissors.

Embryologists say that you are moving more definitely now, Riddle. I like to imagine you kicking your puny legs, waving your fragile arms, nodding your ponderous head to the rhythms of your growth. I like to think of you as an acrobat, turning sedate somersaults in the roomy, weightless chamber of my womb, executing perfectly the maneuvers of your growth while your fingernails sprout, and your jaw fills with the buds that will someday become teeth. I like to imagine you sucking your thumb, curling your toes, stretching your arms, kicking up your heels, simply because you now have a body that can suck, curl, stretch, and kick.

But despite all my imaginings, I cannot feel that dance. My belly is still flat. My guts are not yet aware of the stupendous choreography occurring among them. Intangible, invisible, mute, this baby floats in its amniotic fluid like the future in a crystal ball. The only sign I have of its presence is that for weeks now I have been sick—utterly, wretchedly sick. I gag when I open the refrigerator, and have to turn away from Douglas in bed. Nothing in the world smells wholesome, smells right. Even the smell of my own hair disgusts me. Going to the grocery store is an act of courage. I sleep for hours, wake to retch on a piece of toast, and then stumble back to bed, blank and heavy and miserable.

About morning sickness, both myth and folklore are oddly silent. According to the Bush-ongo of Zaire, the god Bumba created human beings by vomiting them, and I am glad to know that there is a sacred precedent to my misery. I'm glad, too, that at least one father has had to vomit to have children.

The American colonists called it "breeding sickness," which seems an apt name for this nausea that dogs me day and night, and yet, about its causes and cures, they said nothing, noting only what has recently been rediscovered, that a woman who suf-fers with her pregnancy is more likely to give birth to a living, full-term infant than one who does not.

Anthropologists say that morning sickness is culturally conditioned, so that only in those societ-ies where they are expected to feel sick do most women indulge in nausea. Because animals are never ill while they are gestating, psychologists say that morning sickness is an emotional response to the inevitable ambivalence a woman who is newly pregnant feels when she discovers that a condition has been thrust upon her, that, no matter how she has longed for it, will change her life irrevocably. But medical scientists point out that psychological treatments are not effective in curing morning sickness, and say it is really the rich deluge of unfamiliar hormones that can turn a pregnancy into an illness.

It is a mystery, this breeding sickness. Now, as I weep and gag and sleep, I find it easier to understand Eve's curse than the evolution of our species. I feel haunted, invaded, helpless, and then I feel guilty, afraid my longing to be rid of my nausea will rid me of my baby, or will cripple it with some sign of my resentment.

Riddle, you dug yourself into my womb like a cancer or a leech, making yourself at home there like a tapeworm, a flea, a pushy mother-in-law. You commandeered my body, and began complacently growing your own. Long before I was aware of your presence, they say my body was sending white blood cells to try to rid itself of you. And then you set me against myself, for at the same time I was attacking you as though you were an infection, I was also succoring you, sending you the nutrients you needed to survive.

But let me tell you this, little sponge: after Bumba had finished vomiting, he walked through the peaceful villages of his newly disgorged world, telling the people he met, "Behold all these wonders. They are yours." I like to think that I, too, am vomiting to give to you the world's wonders. No matter what it is that makes me ill—my hormones, my culture, or my psyche—still, I am pleased that you have lodged inside me. I am honored by your presence: If you are a parasite, then I am a host—and if I am a host, then you are a welcomed guest.

What wonders you have accomplished, Riddle, as you dance unheeded within me. Already you have all the features that mark you as one of us—vocal cords, opposable thumbs, an upright spine. You have made a gall bladder for yourself, and a pancreas, and a set of kidneys. You have pocked the smooth skin of your face with a pair of eyes, and each eye has sealed itself shut beneath a brand-new lid.

But even though you are blind and deaf, still you have begun to enter the world of sensation. By now you can taste the salty, bitter, and sweet flavors of your amniotic fluid, and your skin is sensitive to its currents. You can feel the tautness of your umbilical cord when you brush against it, and the doubled touch of your own tender self as your hands graze your body. More than two thousand years ago, the philosopher Aristotle said that sensation is the first step on the path that leads from memory to knowledge to wisdom. You're on your way, little Riddle. You're on your way.

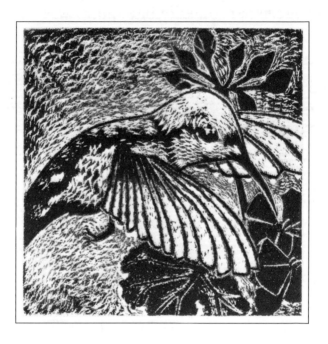

# The Fourth Month

*Woman is the artist of the imagination
and the child in the womb is the canvas
whereon she painteth her pictures.*

### Paracelsus (1493–1541)

For several days I thought they were just the soft rumblings of my own guts, these dim twistings low in my belly. But then one morning as we lay in bed, the twister's father put his hand on my stomach and felt a nudge at the same time I felt a poke. After months of gyrating unobserved, this creature had finally made itself indisputably known, its delicate flutters like a message from a distant planet or a deserted island: Look—there is life here, too! It tapped against its father's palm once more, and then was still, indifferent to the hot blaze of tears in its parents' eyes.

51

## The Life Within

It feels like a kiss, this quickening, like another's tongue slipping and curling inside my mouth. The Eskimos said the aurora borealis was the playing of unborn children. I have seen only the dim, southern version of those northern lights, but still, this sensation is like that, ghostly, lovely, a dance performed in the darkness of another world.

Now as I go about my days, I am aware of the baby brewing inside me, and it surprises me that the pattern of my life is not completely transformed by this quickening. At night, when I lie next to Douglas, I feel the tumbling of the child we have set in motion, and I think I am privy to the mysteries of the goddess. But at other times this tickling in my guts seems usual, normal. Like the passing of gas, or the beating of a heart, it is a familiar feeling, comfortable, homey, and often it comes as no surprise to have this stirring inside me.

I feel newly fond of this old body, now that it is more than just the vehicle of my own continuance. I have forgiven its many curves and softnesses, and I am proud of the neat little bulge of my belly, pleased with my swollen breasts. No longer mine, more than myself, I have become a catalyst, a resource, a puzzle. I am the four-eyed, four-thighed, and forty-nailed beast of the Serbian riddle. I am double-hearted, double-headed, double-tongued. I am a boat rocking an ocean, a basket filling with a single egg. I am a cradle, a crucible, a cauldron, a garden.

'Quicken' means to come to life, and it does seem as though this baby has just begun, now that I can feel its presence. And now that I can distinguish between us, I feel more connection to it than I did before. With these first quiet nudges comes the nascence of love.

In Egypt they say that the heart sees the baby before the eye. But even a heart must be able to see before it can love. Our organs cannot love themselves. Even a heart can only love what is outside of or other than itself, because such a great part of loving is that longing to bridge the distance. Now that it is tangibly separate from me, I find myself asking the lover's question of this finger-length child tucked beneath my heart: Dear Riddle, what is it like for you? They say that already your face, with its newly finished lips, is like no one else's face.

Already the lines that tell your fortune are etched into your tiny palms. Already the whorls have risen on the pads of your fingertips and in the flesh of your feet. What is it like to have that face, those hands and feet?

I wish I could be a twin in your womb, to know what it is you know. I wish I could hear the sounds and silences that your ears have begun to hear, could feel the wash of amniotic fluid on your raw skin. I wish I could learn exactly what this time is like for you. But as I ask those questions to which I know I will never find answers, I learn something else. I learn that imagination is the essence of love.

Today as I drove through town, I passed a white-haired woman struggling up the curb with her walker, and a group of sullen-shouldered teenagers cooling it on a street corner. I passed a pair of plump joggers, and a couple of guys in orange vests working on the road, and suddenly I had a visceral awareness of what logic claims impatiently is obviously so—that we all, every one of us, began as a fluttering in someone else's tummy, amid the guts and goings-on of someone else's life. In that instant of comprehension, I felt the great heave and kick of humanity in the tickle in my belly, and then a maternal tenderness, a mother's indulgent amusement toward the people I drove past.

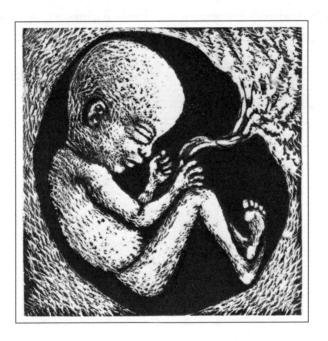

# The Fifth Month

Conception and birth are as stubborn conditions
of life as death itself. Coming to terms
with the rhythms of women's lives
means coming to terms with life itself.

**Margaret Mead**

According to the Thai, pregnancy is like setting out in a little boat to cross an ocean. I am midway through this journey now, and it does sometimes seem as though I were far at sea, with no shore in sight, and only the fertile popple and swell of waves to accompany me toward some uncharted, inevitable land.

My Riddle grows steadily larger. My belly is heaped like a tidy pile of gold, and I catch myself fondling that swelling treasure as though I were a miser. I think I'm as proud of my stomach as if it were my own handiwork, as if I were the potter instead of the bowl.

Yesterday as I was buying groceries, I found myself hefting potatoes, apples, cabbages, pears, weighing them, and then hefting them again, trying to get a sense of the size of the thing I contain. By now this root is as heavy as a turnip, as long as a carrot. Medical photographs show that a twenty-week-old fetus is a porcelain doll of a child, complete with fingernails and eyebrows and a tender fringe of lashes sprouting from the lids of its still-sealed eyes. Fragile, luminous, it seems an unearthly being—more sprite than hearty human—through whose skin shines an intricate lace of veins.

These days I can once again enter a grocery store without retching. My morning sickness, that mundane mystery of this pregnancy, has finally passed. Whether my body has become used to its new flow of hormones, or my psyche has come to terms with the ambivalence of gestation, the nausea has lessened, the exhaustion is gone, and I am once more content to live within my flesh.

Back in the early months of this pregnancy, I felt, for the first time in my life, a great abhorrence

for the fleshliness of living. Everything that had
to do with physicality was disgusting to me. Eating
was a chore, and it seemed these bodies that we were
required constant feeding. The smell of my own
body, of Douglas' body, of the masses of bodies I
passed on the street, made me gag in revulsion. The
sensuality of living, in which I had always reveled,
seemed at best dreary, and at worst, a nightmare. I
understood the monk's longing to be released from
the body, to exist as pure spirit, remote from the
hungers, the rhythms, the filth of the flesh.

I could even begin to understand all those
peoples, from Siberia to the South Pacific, from
Africa to the Far East, who feared the pollution of
pregnancy and birth, as though gestation were the
sort of foul act that Baron Frankenstein committed
when he assembled a living monster from the corp-
ses of the dead. I could almost understand why the
fourth-century Christians began to baptize infants
in the font of waters they called the pure womb of
the church in order to cleanse them of the corrup-
tion of the flesh that bore them.

And I found myself asking if it were true, as
some have claimed, that human flesh is the shape of

all our sorrows, that we are born in suffering, born to suffer. Embryologists say that a fetus' skin grows to cover its growing self in the same way that later its skin will grow to cover its cut fingers or scraped knees. When I was sick and read that, I wondered whether conception itself might be a sort of injury.

I thought of how healing often preserves the form of its hurt, like the bulge in the tree's trunk that hides the ancient noose of wire, or the shiny proud flesh that retains the knife's slash. I remembered other ways in which we are marked forever by our beginnings; the dark line that runs from our navels to our genitals is the remainder of the seam that was formed when we were only the size of apple seeds, and had just begun to sprout symmetrical halves. And I found myself wondering whether our lives were not scarred by their very inceptions, so that, for all their growing, our skins could never heal the stab of suffering at our cores.

But now that I am no longer sick, that sort of thinking once more seems foreign to me. Surely this cycle of fleshiness—messy as it is—is not a dirty thing. The taint of birth is not a universal perception; in the first few days after her baby's delivery, a Jicarilla Apache woman wears her hair unbraided to honor the holiness of her condition—and it seems to me that, given the nature of our lives, we all must celebrate our corporeality. I think of Aristotle's chain linking sensation to wisdom, so that in the end it is our hungry, smelly bodies that make us wise. And I think of the chain that life is, how we were created to create, begotten to beget. The first action of the microscopic bud burgeoning inside me was to set aside those cells that would someday become sperm or ova on their own. Twenty-one days after conception, before the brain, or blood, or lungs are formed, we develop the means to reproduce. Life is that urgent, that insistent upon itself. Before I suspected that I was pregnant, the speck inside me was preparing for my grandchildren.

I think of the body growing in my body, and—if it is female—of the bodies that will grow in it, and of the bodies those unconceived bodies will contain, and I am reminded of a Möbius strip—that clumsy model of infinity—twisting back on itself with each generation...a mother who has a daughter who becomes a mother who has a daughter who becomes a mother...so that there is no beginning, no end, but only this passing through flesh and passing flesh on.

And I think of the other things that travel with flesh, of the touch that has journeyed hand to hand from the beginning, of the wisdom and laughter, the stories and songs that one generation receives from the last, bequeaths to the next. And it seems that flesh is the first gift we must be grateful for.

There is something else that travels with our flesh, something else we pass on: Already this creature wriggling in my womb is practicing its mortality, for it is during this month that the cells it has created start to wear out, to die, to be replaced by others. Already that flesh, that body my Riddle is poised in, is dying, just as mine is, even as it puffs with life.

The Bara of southern Madagascar say that our flesh comes from our mothers and our bone from our fathers. Geneticists have thought that we inherit those blessings equally from both our parents, but recently they have discovered that the

DNA contained in the portion of our cells that produces their energy does not divide and recombine during each new conception as does the DNA of the cell's nucleus. Instead it remains intact, and is passed on entirely by the female to each successive generation. And so it seems possible to trace that mitochondrial DNA back two hundred thousand years to a single woman, an unwitting Eve, through whose womb all of humanity has passed.

I feel a connection to that Cro-Magnon mother now, and to all the mothers who have succeeded her. I sometimes think of us as waves. Grandmother, mother, daughter—each one of us heaves from that moon-driven mass of water, each surges her leagues to shore, there to swell, and roar, and topple into foam, and our lives overlap in the rippled pattern of a single, teaming tide.

I think about fathers, too, these days. Turkish villagers say that we are completely our fathers' children because it is they who plant the seeds of us in the empty fields of our mothers' wombs, but the Trobriand Islanders say that our physical selves come entirely from our mothers, and that if a child grows to resemble its father it is only because of the tender care and nourishment he has given it, both *in utero* and beyond.

According to the Aranda of central Australia, the first human beings were born from their father's armpit as he lay in a swamp of red and purple flowers. Even if subsequent fathers have not given birth to their sons and daughters, still, their role in gestation is a profound one. Medical scientists have discovered many ways in which fathers can affect their unborn children; the baby of an unhappy marriage has a chance of being born damaged that is hundreds of times greater than a baby whose father and mother were in accord before its birth, and even a father's smoking can be detected by the cyanide byproducts in his fetus' blood.

The Arapesh of New Guinea say that childbearing ages a man as much as it does a woman, and the mysterious connection between a father and his unborn has long been recognized throughout the world with customs of couvade, in which fathers, too, have had to endure certain restrictions in order to ensure the life and health of their coming children. An expectant Chinese father must always move gently so that his womb-child will not be hurt by the violence of his actions, and a Malay father may not kill anything lest that cruelty damage his fetus. A Bagesu father must walk carefully, because if he were to fall, his baby might be miscarried, and a Nicobarese father cannot tie a rope, for fear the spirit of his unborn will be caught in the knot.

A Kamchatkan father must not do heavy work, a father in New Guinea may not chew betel, a father in the Solomon Islands must not eat pork. In the New Hebrides, an expectant father may not enter sacred places, and in the North Celebes, he must not sit with his legs crossed. A Dayak father can't light fires, a Jambim father can't fish, and a Philippine father can't eat sour fruit—all so that the babies those fathers have engendered will be born whole and hale and with a chance of happiness.

But perhaps neither fatherhood nor motherhood matter all that much. The Australian Aborigines thought that every baby was the incarnation of a tribal ancestor, a being much older than anyone living at the time of its birth. Because each infant was so ancient, the Aborigines believed there was no biological bond between parents and their children. Each baby was an independent entity who might have easily been the offspring of any other woman. A mother only incubated whatever spirit-child chose to reside inside her, and the resulting baby was a human being no more hers than any other human being would be.

While my mother was birthing my brother, my father drank sour coffee and paced the hospital halls, as fathers in the nineteen-fifties were supposed to do. When a nurse finally arrived to tell him he had a son, he grinned, said, "That's wonderful!" and asked her, "What's his name?"

I know that embedded in his gentle joke was my father's conviction that a child arrives in its parents' lives so entire, so completely and uniquely itself that it is a surprise it does not come named. Children are no more ours than rivers or clouds, no more ours than even our own borrowed flesh, which we must some day return to the earth. We do not own, cannot possess our children, and instead of "having" this baby, perhaps its father and I should think of "giving" it.

These days I am aware that when I touch my swollen belly, it is not me I am feeling, not my own flesh I caress, but the thing that flips and wiggles and rests against the pressure of my palm.

And so, I stroke my own taut skin, and dream of the child my flesh conceals. I have grown impatient to meet it, to trace its rubbery features, to cup its soft-fisted hands, to rock it, and suckle it, and share my world with it. I want to show it all I love, the iridescent hummingbirds darting among the red geraniums, the stars droning like crickets in the night sky. I want it with me now, to hear the fragile rain, to smell the green earth, to watch the oak leaves dance as the raindrops hit them. I am doubly aware of the world these days; I hear and smell and see and touch and taste it twice—once for myself, and once for this Riddle who has not yet known a summer rain.

But what could this root possibly know of my world? I rub the dumb bulk of my stomach and wonder when and how consciousness comes to inhabit the body my body harbors. It might be that it precedes fertilization as some sort of racial memory in the nucleic acids of the chromosomes themselves, or that it ignites in the moment of fusion, when the chromosomes find their partners, and the two cells become one—though when I consider those possibilities, when I try to imagine the awareness of hormones and proteins, or the cognizance of uniting chromosomes, my mind reels and can find no imagery for such things.

Maybe consciousness arrives later—on the eighteenth day, with the foundations of the nervous system; during the third month, with the first brain waves; or during the eighth month, with the coming of dreams. Or it could be that consciousness emerges with something to be conscious of, so that it develops gradually, as the senses develop—first touch and taste, now hearing, and finally sight and smell, all serving to fuel the spark inside me.

Or maybe those Victorians were right, who said that a baby knew nothing until long after its birth. Maybe the thing inside me is still as blank as a tulip bulb, simply sprouting, budding, blooming, because that is what bulbs do when there is water and soil and light and heat enough to permit their growth.

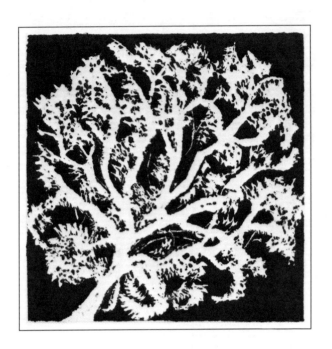

# The Sixth Month

*The woman conceives. As a mother she is another person than the woman without child. She carries the fruit of the night for nine months in her body. Something grows. Something grows into her life that never again departs from it. She is a mother. She is and remains a mother even though her child dies, though all her children die. For at one time she carried the child under her heart. And it does not go out of her heart ever again.*

**An Abyssinian Woman**

The Siamese say that a six-month-old fetus is like a monkey huddled in the rain, trying to warm itself at the base of a tree. The photographs show that this baby is now achingly skinny, with short, squatting legs and a delicate fur. Because it has an inhumanly powerful grip, and more taste buds than it will have when it is born, embryologists say that it still retains some connections with its simian past, connections it will lose in the next sixteen weeks as it grows towards its *Homo sapiens* future.

71

They say, too, that its brain is as smooth now as a monkey's brain, without the furrows that will one day mark it as one of ours.

Little monkey, you must use these next few months to get fat and smart. You must grow fat enough so that you can shed your fur, and still bear the cold of the coming world. And your smooth egg of a brain must grow convoluted—complex and diverse enough to allow you to reason, to question, to juggle symbols and apples. You must abandon your instincts, little chimp. You must forsake the reflex that allowed your ancestors to cling to their mothers' fur as they swung through the green tangle of forest, and you must take up instead the rich jungle of your own wrinkled brain.

This ape has begun to crowd itself out of the freedom it once knew. No longer can it leap and somersault in an ecstasy of weightlessness. Now it is bound by the flesh that contains it, bound by its own flesh, so that wherever it squirms, it bumps against its elbows or knees, or the arch of its mother's ribs.

## The Sixth Month

We can't escape each other. Always when it moves I know it now. It pummels my kidneys, kicks my stomach, punches my lungs. I know when it is resting, and when it wakes and stretches. I know it well by now. I, who have never before had a baby move inside me, tell its father it will be a calm, a happy child.

It knows me, too. It dangles upside down inside me like a bat, listening to all my doings. Its sealed eyes have opened, uncovering retinas capable of transforming light to image, but they show it only the shadowy closeness of my womb. It cannot yet smell, can taste only the waters that surround it, can feel only its own slippery body. The world those senses show it is a muffled place, bland and unchanging. Still, that mild space is filled with noise, with the harmonies, cacophonies, and silences of its mother's life.

It hears all that I hear, the sounds intensified and distorted like the disembodied, directionless racket one hears under the water in a swimming pool. It hears, too, the busy workings of my body, the burble of my intestines, the air breezing in my lungs. It hears the gust of my farts, the rumble of

73

my burps, the gulp each time I swallow. And always, always it hears the cozy beating of my heart.

Leonardo Da Vinci thought that because the same body nourished both mother and fetus, then the same soul must also sustain them both. But in Bang Chan it was said that a pregnant woman was double-souled, and so strong was the power of those twinned souls that if she died before giving birth, her fetus would have to be cut from her body so that the living would be free of the threat of a two-souled ghost.

Single- or double-souled, it is a strange sense of oneness and duality I feel these days. I know the flesh I grow is grown from my flesh, and that what I eat now nourishes not only me, but the body within my body. And I know of other, more subtle connections that would seem to make us one beast. Scientists say that even before a woman who smokes lights her cigaret, her fetus' heartbeat will increase. And they are beginning to believe what folklore has claimed for thousands of years, that a woman's worries or joys may be translated into hormones that can affect her developing child.

## The Sixth Month

This fetus and I share even the chemistry of my emotions, so wholly are we joined, but within my sense of unity is the uncanny feeling that I am now two entities. At this moment in my very womb, there are hands feeling what I will never feel, a mind beginning its solitary comprehension. I now embody something as distinct from me, as vastly distant from me, as another human being. Beloved as it is, it is a stranger that I nourish.

This morning I sat outside, sipping tea and dreaming while the stranger in me slept. As I drowsed in the warm drench of autumn sunlight, I remembered how the people of Mali once believed the sun was the placenta of the first human being. I lifted my shirt, and eased my pants down over the mute, white mountain of my belly, so that Riddle, too, might absorb its share of light. Suddenly it stirred, seemed to stretch, and my whole stomach shifted and heaved with its waking.

I lifted my face to the sun, closed my eyes, and saw the red haze of light seeping through my shut lids. I thought that perhaps, with its newly opened eyes, the kitten my Riddle is was seeing something similar as the sun filtered through my skin and muscle to flood the chamber of my womb. I imagined Riddle bathed in silent, blood-colored light. I was pleased that the color of the sun through its mother's flesh was the first color it would know, and I wondered when each of us first became capable of awe.

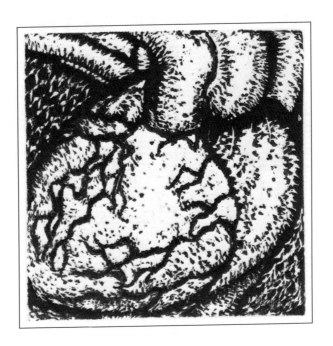

# The Seventh Month

*Man is the only one that knows nothing, that can
learn nothing without being taught. He can neither
speak nor walk nor eat, and in short he can do nothing
at the prompting of nature only, but weep.*

**Pliny the Elder (AD 23-79)**

Medical researchers say that memory begins
during the seventh month, for now this baby's brain
is beginning to lose its apple-smoothness, and become rutted, capable of storing the impressions of
its experience. I think of those memories like the
first fragile tracks on a newly fallen snow—delicate
bird-prints, perhaps, or maybe simply the preserved
shape of the wind—where later will come larger,
more definite patterns, where later trails will be
worn, paths that connect and shape what was once
a single expanse of whiteness.

I wonder what this child will remember of
this moment, this afternoon in early autumn, as I sit

at my desk and look out the window to the slow, green river. A yellow leaf drops from the oak tree and twirls to the water's surface. A blue jay squawks from the roof. The typewriter drones its soothing, electrical hum, and when I type, the keys clatter like a fistful of pebbles tossed on a stony beach. Perhaps the baby sleeps, and this moment is nothing more than the vague chatter of my typing and the steady beating of our hearts. Or perhaps it is awake, wondering at the miracle taking place inside its skull as it hears my typing and ferrets it away, hiding it in its blank brain like a squirrel hiding a nut it may never find again.

I canned applesauce this morning. Resting my belly against the counter, I quartered and cored a bushel of Jonathans, and tossed the pieces into the old soup kettle on the stove. For a while the baby thumped companionably inside me, and then it grew still, leaving me to my solitary work and thought.

As I cut apples, I remembered how as a child I had once been shown that if you sliced an apple not from the stem end down, but straight through its middle, there, etched into the center of each half would be a flower whose five petals sheathed the seeds that could grow new trees. I remember being charmed by that chicken-or-eggish puzzle: The apple came from a flower and contained a flower, in an infinite regression of fruitfulness.

This morning, while I stirred the fragrant kettle, I thought how the apples steaming beneath my spoon might feed the Riddle napping in my stomach. I thought of all the other preparations that had been made for this new flower, how seeds had been planted, rains had fallen, fruit had been harvested to satisfy an appetite still unborn, and I remembered that the Melpa of New Guinea had said that a baby's afterbirth must always be buried so that that which once connected it to its mother could now connect it to the earth.

I washed canning jars in soapy water and thought how thoroughly we are wedded to this earth, from before our births to beyond our deaths. I remembered the loaf of homemade bread that I chanced upon in my mother's kitchen after my father's sudden death. It was a loaf my father had baked himself, a loaf risen to the shape of his hands, and that loaf sustained me long after the last crumbs had been swallowed.

As I filled the scalded jars with thick, hot pulp, I marveled at how even a bit of bread or a bowl of applesauce can link our lives to lives beyond ours in the grave or womb. And then, as my hands worked and my mind wandered, the secret flower at an apple's core reminded me of a star, and I remembered a time last summer, when this heft of baby was just a tickle in my flat stomach, and my brother showed me the night sky through his telescope. First we looked at Jupiter's split rings, at Mars' red stripe, at the jewel that is Venus. Then he pointed the telescope into the emptiness above our infinitesimal heads, and adjusted the lens again. I bent, squinted into the eyepiece, and saw something more marvelous than even the planets of my solar system, saw a tiny smudge of light like a mote of dust in a hay barn in late afternoon.

"The Andromeda Galaxy," he said, "That light is two million years old." I gazed at that ancient blur, felt the baby glimmer in my stomach, and thought not of distances and isolation, but of connections. I thought how we were constructed of the same elements blazing in that infinity of stars, and I wondered at all that had existed between the instant that light left its galaxy and the moment that I witnessed it. I thought then, as I think now, how rich and vast our lives are, that connect both apples and stars.

Riddle, if you were born now, you would gasp at the air like a landed fish, and yet there is a chance those water-logged sponges that are your lungs could glean enough oxygen for you to survive. Of all our organs, our lungs are said to be most like other mammals', but even so, our lungs give us an ability few other creatures possess, for when we can breathe, we can also weep. In rural Japan it was thought an infant's first cry was evidence a human spirit had entered its nonhuman body; if a fetus were stillborn, or if it died without crying, then it had never been a human being. So it may be that our ability to cry is another of the things that makes us human.

I wish I could tell you more clearly what it means, to be human. I think it is important. I think it is a privilege to be a keeper of language, a maker of symbol, to have hands that can shape what our minds can imagine. I think it is a privilege to be able to love, even in the clumsy ways we humans love.

But strengths are always weaknesses, and so, as humans, we are doomed by the language we have created to feel isolated from all that surrounds us, doomed by our ability to think in symbols to hunger for meaning, doomed by our agility as tool-makers to make monstrosities. Being human is a strange thing, unsettling, uncomfortable—at times unbearable. You'll suffer your humanity, Riddle. You'll writhe in the face of your limitations and your losses. You'll ache with grief and rage and uncertainty, and still your life will flow on, unbidden, out of your control.

Perhaps that is why we who have already cried sometimes long to occupy the place where the unborn live, why we want to return to the womb where we can be warm and weightless once again, where we can be nourished without having to eat, be loved without being touched. But still, few of us would ever give up our places among the born and breathing. Even when we are suffering most profoundly, when we are standing over fresh graves, or when our lives are filled with terror, boredom, or despair, even as we weep, we share with those who are not yet born the vigorous urge to live.

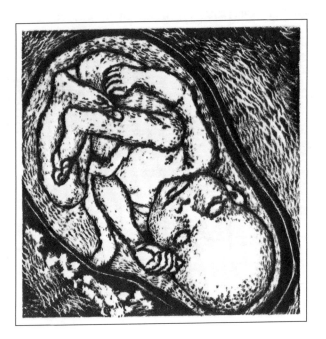

# The Eighth Month

*I'm a means, a stage, a cow in calf.*
*I've eaten a bag of green apples,*
*Boarded the train there's no getting off.*

**Sylvia Plath**

The ancient Egyptians called their goddess of pregnancy and childbirth Ta-urt, The Great One, and it is thought that even when they revered her she was old, harkening back to some primeval time when birth was the sole religion, and she the only deity. In their art the Egyptians portrayed her as a rampant hippopotamus, rearing back on her hind legs to reveal her distended stomach and huge, hanging breasts. She is ferocious, ridiculous, enormously gravid, The Great One through whose fecund body we all must pass.

I feel akin to that pregnant goddess, now
that my feet have been eclipsed by my full moon
of a belly, my waist swallowed by this watermelon
that swells majestically in front of me. When I
examine myself in the mirror, I feel a strange mixture of horror and complacent pride; my ballooning
stomach is absurd, grotesque, stunningly lovely—a
surprising globe thrusting itself into the world.

My breasts, too, have grown. Heavy, full,
they bulge above my bulging stomach, each crowned
with a nipple so startlingly thick that I wonder how
it will ever fit in a newborn's mouth. They leak a
little now and then, the colostrum that already
adapts itself to this Riddle's growth, so that even if
it were born prematurely, the milk it drank would be
precisely suited to its needs.

In Kenya, the Gusii word for 'birthing' also
means 'to nurse,' as though birthing and suckling
were no more divisible than the press and release of
a single kiss, and there are English words whose
histories also reveal something about what it means
to suckle a child. Our word 'galaxy' is a remnant of
the Greek word for milk, because the Greeks said
that it was milk spraying from the goddess Hera's

breasts that created the stars of the Milky Way. A seventeenth-century meaning of 'blithe' was 'yielding milk,' and I like to think of my breasts as blithe, able to yield a merry, milky joy to the baby who rises beneath them.

The villagers of Sri Lanka believe that human milk is blood that has been heated and purified in a woman's body, but scientists say that milk is actually sweat, modified with fats, proteins, sugars, vitamins, and minerals, and enriched with antibodies that can protect an infant from allergies and colds and cancers. They say that of all mammals, humans produce the sweetest milk, and, because one of the molecules of milk sugar also makes up most of the gray matter of our brains, they speculate that it is the sweetness of our mothers' milk that makes us smart.

It is said that the first baptisms were performed when a woman exercised her right of name-giving by squirting her infant with her milk as she spoke its name, and it does seem as though it were holy stuff. I sometimes think of my milk-to-come as a kind of Eucharist—no grim and glorious sacrifice, but an easy, cozy, female blessing of body and blood.

Riddle, back when you were a blastocyst, and I was no more aware of you than I am of the yet-undiscovered galaxies that speckle the reaches of our universe, your father and I took to the ocean one day to watch for migrating whales. Over and over our boat rose and tipped and sank with the slaty swells, and now and then we caught sight of the mass of a whale's back mounting from the water. Each time we watched breathless as it spewed a chill torrent from its blowhole, and then slid back into the depths, vanishing finally with a fillip of its flukes. It seemed to us as if mountains were dancing, or as if the coastal redwoods had taken to cavorting in the sea.

Once during that afternoon, we watched a gray whale suckle her calf. From where we stood on the rocking boat, it was no great spectacle; she rolled on her side so that only one huge fin broke the water, and her calf submerged itself beside her for a second. Then they both blew and sounded, and we were left alone on the pitching deck to wonder at what we had seen.

## The Eighth Month

Sometimes when it moves now, this baby seems like a whale, surging up from the deeps to romp and blow before it sounds again its airless fathoms. At other times it seems to move like the slow heave of the whole ocean, whose dense waters conceal tiny, lively secrets—the quick trickle in the veins, the sea horse heart.

So much have I been distorted by this pregnancy that my own heart now lies beating sideways on top of my uterus, and my guts, lungs, and bladder have all been squeezed out of its way. It is hard to be this great-bellied, hard to have to lug this flour sack of a stomach with me wherever I go. I pant even when I'm resting, and have to pee constantly. I long to be able to run, to bound out of bed, to take the stairs by twos. Instead, I collapse into chairs, and have to heave myself to my feet again. I can't sleep, can't bend, can hardly tie my shoes. I am slow, ponderous, burdened with this baby.

But to have a flat stomach, roomy and empty except for the private twistings of my own intestines, seems a meager existence now. I cannot remember what it was like to have my guts to myself, to live without this thumping and sleeping inside me. I will miss this burgeoning when it has left me, will miss this drowsy feeling of fecundity, and the heavy stretch of my skin.

The Arapesh say that a baby sleeps until it it awoken by its birth, but neurologists claim that by the eighth month this fetus will have begun a cycle of waking and sleeping whose rhythms are already influenced by the sun. And they say that when it sleeps, it dreams—or at least its brain waves resemble those of a dreamer. I know that it is impossible to share the dreams even of those who share my world, but still I find myself wondering what this sleeper dreams.

Little Riddle, are your dreams bounded by your experience, so that they consist only of the echo of my voice, the remembered motion of your body, the feel of the womb reenacted inside your head? Or do your dreams already take you inside yourself, beyond yourself? Do your dreams remind you of what it was you left behind when you entered the realm of protoplasm, so that your sleep is filled with the memories of your race, memories of the heroes and deeds of four million years of human history? Or do your dreams take you beyond that heritage, back to a time when you loped over the savannah, frolicked in an empty sea, or warmed yourself on a stone that has long since turned to dust?

Maybe you dream the course of your growth, of splitting cells, of branching veins, of nerves groping to connect. Or perhaps you dream of the time when you will be aquatic no longer, when your lungs will expand like birthday party balloons, and your own voice will croak in your throat. Do you dream of the feel of arms that are not your own, of the fit of a nipple in your mouth, and the stretch of your belly filled with milk? Or is the world that fills your dreams a rosy place, rich with the murmur of blood, and the beat of a heart like a sun overhead, a utopia of the unborn, inhabited by a race of silent swimmers like yourself whose hollow stomachs never ache for food, whose flat lungs never grope for air, whose empty hands never yearn for other hands to hold?

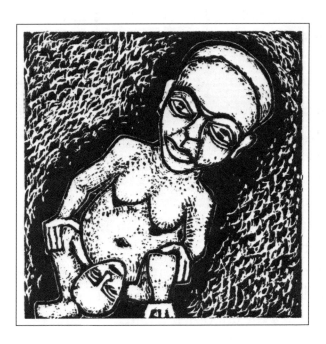

# The Ninth Month

*A birth is a birth, and any human birth is the same*
*as any other. It is anonymous, in short,*
*and it might be said to be the birth of somebody supreme*
*in the land of lore and legend, the son of God,*
*that is to say, or the daughter of Heaven,*
*and the mother might be said to be the mother of God.*

**William Saroyan**

This jail-bird is a short-termer now. Its life
beyond the bars of my ribs looms ahead, and I
think it begins to long for that freedom, even
though out here it will be trapped yet again, not by
the closeness of its cell, but by its sudden needs for
heat and food and air.

As it serves the last days of its sentence, it
makes the final preparations for its escape. It spends
most of its time sucking amniotic fluid in and out of
its lungs, to strengthen them for their first and
hardest breath, when they must inflate even the

tiny air sacs in their stiff walls. It is growing plumper, too, padding the rind of itself against the coming cold, provisioning itself for its abrupt weaning from my blood, when it must live off its own stores of fat until my milk comes in.

But I know that despite all its arrangements, this baby will enter the world just half gestated, born now only because if it were not, its burgeoning head could never squeeze through the girdle of my pelvic bones; it will be another nine months before this possum is as fully developed as other primates are when they are born. And so I am reminded of the arbitrariness of birth—in the years to come, when we celebrate this Riddle's birthday, there is a way in which we will be commemorating little more than a change in its means of respiration and nutrition.

Turkish villagers give bawdy encouragement to a woman nearing term by telling her, "May the baby come out as easily as it went in." But in India, a woman who loses courage in the throes of her labor will be scolded by her midwife, who demands "What baby was ever born without pain?" In Denmark, it was said that a woman could secure a pain-

less labor for herself if she would stretch a foal's caul
between four sticks and crawl beneath it, but the
price she paid for doing so was that her sons would
be born werewolves and her daughters night hags.
And so—by choice or not—we suffer in childbirth,
and whether that pain is thought of as being caused
by evil spirits, a god's curse, a woman's fears, or
simply the straining of her cervix depends on the
culture in which we labor.

There are cultures in which fathers, too,
must endure the pain of birth. Some are said to do
so because they have been tricked by their wives, as
the Scottish groom who made the mistake of rising
before his bride on the first morning of their marriage. But other fathers have suffered voluntarily,
because they believed that their anguish would ease
the pain their wives felt, and so the native men of
New Ireland and North India and Central Califor-
nia would take to their beds, and there writhe in the
torment of labor as their children were being born.

Elsewhere, men have acted in other ways as
their women were birthing. On Easter Island, it is
the father himself who must deliver his child, but in
the Pacific Islands, a father must wait in seclusion

until his baby has arrived. In Central Africa, a father may be bathed by his sister-in-law if his wife's contractions slow, while in Eastern Africa, a father might dig certain roots for his mate to chew in order to hasten her labor.

Scientists say that labor helps an infant adapt to its postnatal life, that the adrenaline it receives from its mother sends extra blood to its vital organs, and produces the chemicals that will ease the inflation of its lungs. During labor, the uterus, which has become a muscle temporarily stronger than even a heart, must stretch the cervix at its base from an opening the circumference of a mustard seed to something that could encompass a grapefruit. Because it is much less painful to be squeezed than it is to be stretched, they say a birthing baby may feel nothing more than the pressure of its familiar waters while contractions rack its mother. For a baby, contractions may be caresses that express the fluid from its lungs and stimulate its skin in the same way that other mammals, with their shorter labors, do by licking their newborns.

When I try to imagine what this labor will be like, my imagination loses itself in a fog as abrupt and impenetrable as the fog that shrouds my death. I can envision my life up until the moment that my contractions begin, and then the images become feeble, vague cliches: I do not know what it means, to have a baby. I've tried to imagine reaching between my legs to feel, in that most private place, flesh that isn't mine. I've tried to imagine the slimy bulge of another's head opening from me like an eye, and then that head crowning—regally purple —out of me, tried to imagine that sudden creature in my arms, but always the vision slithers away, and I am left empty-armed, unopened, waiting.

I think when we finally see each other, we will be like two old friends, pen pals from distant countries, who began writing as children, and who understand each other through their letters better than lovers, but who might pass on the street without a glance. I think we will recognize each other blindly, by touch and sniff, as animals do. We know each other from the inside out, this baby and I, who must part to meet.

And now I am moved by all the ways there are for a woman to give birth. I think of the Navaho woman who delivers amidst a happy crowd of friends and family, of the Gilyak woman who must leave her home, even in a storm, to give birth in a hut so crude it cannot shelter her from the cold and wind, of the Yukaghir woman whose father holds her as she delivers his grandchild, of the Japanese peasant who must labor in silence, because to moan would be to shame herself. It seems each of those births says something different, something important and profound about who we women are and what our lives can mean.

But I think the births that move me most are those in which women, either through convention or necessity, must face their labors alone. The !Kung Bushmen of Botswana, the Seneca Indians of North America, the Chukchee of Siberia, all believe a woman should endure her labor and deliver her child unaided. And so it would seem that one thing childbirth can be is an act so simple that nothing more is needed than the blanket a woman carries with her as she slips from the village. Or perhaps it is that the birth of a baby can be a coming to terms with oneself, a discovery of the courage, endurance, knowledge, and faith that, through instinct or grace, can be a woman's birthright.

I once read a journal kept by an American woman in the 1920s, who, because of foul weather and bad luck, was stranded alone for a winter in a tiny cabin in eastern Alaska. There, after two days of solitary labor, she gave birth to a daughter, and although in her diary she writes not of her own accomplishment, but of her newborn child, still, I am both thrilled and humbled when I consider what she must have suffered, and what she must have learned during those lonely hours of birthing.

It may be that laboring alone embodies a reality of all labors, for no matter how many and how beloved their birth attendants, perhaps finally all women must face themselves and the inescapable conditions of their bodies and their lives as they labor for their babies. Perhaps in childbirth, as in death, we are confronted most clearly with the essential aloneness of our existence.

And yet when we labor we are never alone, for birth, like sex, is a dance for two. A woman in labor is flooded with the same hormones that surge through her body during sex; her uterus contracts in a similar way; at times even her voice and face might be the voice and face of a woman making love. In childbirth, too, she must both surrender to the urgencies of another, and follow the dictates of her own body until that path leads her beyond herself, to something she could not have found alone.

The Egyptian hieroglyphic for 'to give birth to' is a squatting woman with an upside-down head emerging from her genitals. The oldest sculptures I have seen are the blunt stone carvings of women from between whose unabashed and powerful thighs a second head pokes, and I love the absurdity, the mystery, the matter-of-fact female glory of those double-headed goddesses.

When the Lapp women of the last century gave birth, they were thought to be under the protection of Sarakka, the Creator-woman. The ancient Babylonians said that it was Ninhursag who bore humankind, and in their birthing chants they evoked her name, for they believed that every woman reenacts Ninhursag's sacred birth as she labors. I find myself remembering those forgotten goddesses as my own time draws near. I think of them as a single woman, the mother of us all, who, frightened by the cramp in her bloated womb, sought the safest place she knew, and there hunkered into herself to heal or die.

For hours, the mosses below her, the trees and stars above, widened, dimmed, spun with her pain, until I imagine she did what I am told that all laboring women must do—she abandoned her life, gave herself up to the rhythms of the world, the inexorable push of water, the implacable grind of stone, the ache and grip of her womb.

Finally, when she could no longer help it, she squatted over her labor, began to push, her dark vulva bulging with the shape of a living head, her self opening like a scream. For an instant she was two-headed, and then a human being slithered from her, plopped breathing on the blood-soaked moss. And when she rose with that infant in her arms, her face was serene as the face of the goddesses she became.

And now all custom, all folk wisdom, seems to forget its wishes for a whole and healthy child, and to concern itself only with the tricks and prayers and charms that will help a woman expel her fetus before she dies. It's a risky time, this reckoning, a time when a woman may lose her soul, if not her life. The heaven the Aztecs inhabited when they died was red with the blood of their heroes—the men who were killed in battle, and the women who were killed in childbirth. The Bariba of West Africa said that a pregnant woman was a dying woman, and two hundred years ago, when one of every fifteen women perished in childbirth, Puritan women were told to prepare for Paradise as their earthly travail drew near. In all places, at all times, birth has carried with it the threat of death, and people have done whatever they could to deliver their women safely.

In India and Ireland, Siberia and the Americas, and among the wandering Gypsies, the whole of an expectant woman's house and life becomes metaphor for her labor, and so doors must be opened, hair loosened, pots uncovered, animals set free, all so that there will be no obstructions or hesitations when she gives birth. Elsewhere a pregnant woman may not tell lies, drive nails, or kill animals because her actions might slow her infant's coming. When she is walking, she must not turn back for fear that during her delivery, her baby will do the same. Even words like 'stuck' or 'fastened' are sometimes taboo lest they define the progress of a woman's labor.

I have read about labors that lasted for two days, four days, nine days, only to end in the woman's dying undelivered, or in delivering, and then dying—of a ruptured uterus, or hemorrhage, or childbed fever. I have read of the brutality of embryotomy, the agony of version, of women who were beaten, poisoned, bled, or abandoned when their labors went wrong, and I am grateful that I am pregnant in this time, when I do not risk my life to deliver my child.

But even though I know I will survive this pregnancy, I feel as though I were approaching something akin to death as my time draws near. I am helpless in the face of this impending labor; at some unknown moment a process will begin in my very body that I can neither imagine nor control, and from that time on, the life I am leading now will be gone forever.

Some would say it is the hidden memory of my own birth that makes me think of death as this birth draws near. They would claim the fetus in the womb lives in an Atlantis, a Utopia, an Eden of bliss, until suddenly that perfect world turns hostile, its foundations heave, and that innocent princeling is thrust from grace, battered and squeezed through an impossible passage, only to emerge at last, bruised and exhausted, a foundling in a place of dry confusion and unfiltered sound.

It is said we fear death because we dread having to relive the ordeal that was our birth, that hidden in our worst nightmares are the terrors we learned aborning. Newborn puppies have sometimes been seen to turn back, to battle blindly past their lolling, gooey wombmates, in a desperate attempt to reenter that tunnel, to gain again the asylum of the womb. Even with their eyes sealed, even with the warm lash of their bitch's tongue and the promise of her milk they know the world is both too meager and too much, and they would forsake it all for what they just struggled to leave.

But if entering this world is a kind of death, how much more deadly must the womb become, for there we are buried, crowded in upon ourselves, isolated from our senses, always alone. Europeans in the Middle Ages thought that an infant procured its own delivery by kicking itself from the womb. Today medical scientists echo that belief when they say it is not the mother, but the fetus, who produces the hormones that begin labor. And I wonder if this baby lurching inside me doesn't long to get on with it, to abandon the womb, to live, even—if its birth requires it—to die.

•

The ancient Mayan year consisted of 260 days, a number that corresponds with neither the seasons nor the stars, but with the length of human gestation. According to our calendar, which measures time by the orbits and rotations of the earth, it takes three-quarters of a year—thirty-eight weeks—nine and a half months—for a human being to travel from its conception to its birth, turning from a single cell into something six billion times as large, and so vast, so complex that even its own understanding will never be able to grasp all that it is.

Time passes strangely for us these last two weeks. There are moments when this baby thrashes inside me as though it could bear its confinement no longer, as though movement alone could free it, but then it will still, floating immobile in its eternal waters, until I get lonely, and have to tap my stomach to rouse it and feel it move.

I, too, alternate between impatience and passivity. At times I rush about in a flurry of hot water and soap, preparing our house to receive this guest, and then I will sit cat-slow for hours, watching the colorless rain slant into the river, and the fire flicker in the stove, drowsing, dreaming of nothing but the slow pull of the rain, the red pulse of the flame.

And so we wait, poised between our two worlds, until the waiting seems stable, fixed, as though we would remain forever in these hugely pregnant days. Then the waiting ceases, the goal fades, and our being, this moment of fire and water and rich flesh, is all there is.

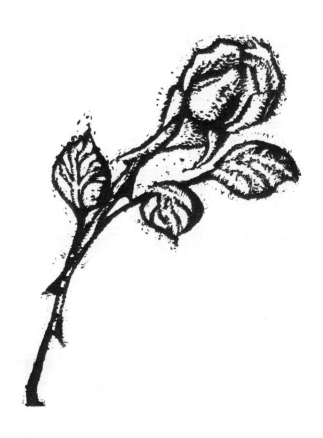